How to Boost Immune System Naturally

The Ultimate Guide to Preventing and Treating Common Illnesses

DR. J. K. EVANS

Table of content

Introduction

What is the immune system and why is it important?

Which components influence the immune system?

What are the benefits of having a strong immune system?

How can natural remedies help boost the immune system?

Chapter 1: Nutrition and Immunity

How does nutrition influence the immune system?

What are the essential nutrients for immune health?

What are the best foods to eat to boost the immune system?

What are the foods to avoid or limit to prevent immune suppression?

Chapter 2: Herbs and Supplements for Immunity

How do herbs and supplements support the immune system?

What are the most effective herbs and supplements for immune health?

How to use herbs and supplements safely and effectively?

What are the possible interactions and side effects of herbs and supplements?

Here are some examples of herbs and supplements that can interact with medicines:

Chapter 3: Lifestyle and Immunity

How does lifestyle affect the immune system?

Some of the lifestyle factors that can influence the immune system are:

What are the best practices to enhance the immune system?

How to manage stress, sleep, exercise, and hygiene for immune health?

How to avoid or reduce exposure to toxins and pathogens that weaken the immune system.

To avoid or reduce exposure to toxins and pathogens that weaken the immune system, here are some tips to follow:

Chapter 4: Natural Remedies for Common Immune Disorders

Natural Remedies for Common Immune Disorders

What are the common immune disorders and their causes and symptoms?

How to Prevent and Treat Common Immune Disorders Naturally

Natural Remedies for Colds, Flu, Allergies, Asthma, Autoimmune Diseases, and More

When to Seek Medical Help and What are the Conventional Treatments for Immune Disorders

When to Seek Medical Help

What are the Conventional Treatments

Conclusion

A summary of the main points and key takeaways from the book

Here are some ways you can start implementing these natural strategies today:

A list of additional resources and references for further reading and learning

To leave a review, you can follow these steps:

Introduction

What is the immune system and why is it important?

The immune system is a complex network of cells, tissues, organs, and molecules that protects the body from harmful invaders, such as bacteria, viruses, parasites, and toxins. The immune system is essential for our survival, as it helps us fight infections and diseases, and also maintains our overall health and well-being.

There are two main kinds of immune systems in our body: the innate immune system and the adaptive immune system. The innate immune system is the first line of defense, and it responds quickly and broadly to any foreign substance or organism. The innate immune system includes physical barriers (such as skin and mucous membranes), chemical barriers (such as saliva and stomach acid), and cellular components (such as natural killer cells and macrophages).

The adaptive immune system is the second line of defense, and it responds more slowly and specifically to a particular antigen. The adaptive immune system involves the production of antibodies and memory cells, which can recognize and eliminate the same antigen in the future.

The immune system is important because it helps us prevent and recover from infections and diseases, which can otherwise cause serious harm or even death. The immune system also plays a role in other aspects of our health, such as wound healing, inflammation, allergy, autoimmunity, and cancer. A healthy immune system can balance the immune responses and avoid excessive or inappropriate reactions that can damage the body's own tissues. Therefore, it is vital to take care of our immune system and support its optimal functioning.

Which components influence the immune system?

The immune system is influenced by many factors, both internal and external, that can either enhance or impair its function. Some of the factors that affect the immune system are:

Age: The immune system changes with age, and it tends to decline as we get older. This makes us more susceptible to infections and diseases, and also reduces the effectiveness of vaccines and medications. However, some aspects of the immune system, such as memory cells and antibodies, can improve with age and experience .

Genetics: The immune system is partly inherited from our parents, and it varies among individuals and populations. Some people have genetic mutations or variations that make them more or less prone to certain immune disorders, such as allergies, autoimmune diseases, or immunodeficiencies .

Stress: Stress can have both positive and negative effects on the immune system, depending on the type, duration, and intensity of the stressor. Short-term stress can boost the immune system by activating the fight-or-flight response, which increases the production of adrenaline and cortisol. However, chronic or long-term stress can suppress the immune system by reducing the number and activity of immune cells, and increasing the risk of inflammation and infection .

Sleep: Sleep is essential for the immune system, as it helps to regulate the circadian rhythm, which affects the production and release of immune cells and molecules. Lack of sleep or poor quality sleep can impair the immune system by reducing the number and function of natural killer cells, T cells, and B cells, and increasing the levels of pro-inflammatory cytokines. This can make us more vulnerable to infections and diseases, and also affect the response to vaccines and treatments .

Exercise: Exercise can have both positive and negative effects on the immune system, depending on the frequency, intensity, and duration of the physical activity. Moderate exercise can enhance the immune system by increasing the circulation of immune cells, improving the lymphatic system, and reducing stress and inflammation. However, excessive or strenuous exercise can suppress the immune system by causing tissue damage, increasing cortisol levels, and depleting energy and nutrients .

Diet: Diet can have a significant impact on the immune system, as it provides the nutrients and energy that the immune cells need to function properly. A balanced diet that includes a variety of fruits, vegetables, whole grains, lean proteins, healthy fats, and probiotics can boost the immune system by providing antioxidants, vitamins, minerals, and other phytochemicals that can modulate the immune responses and protect against oxidative stress and inflammation. However, a poor diet that is high in processed foods, refined sugars, saturated fats, and alcohol can impair the immune system by causing nutrient deficiencies, dysbiosis, obesity, and metabolic disorders .

Environment: The environment can also affect the immune system, as it exposes us to various factors that can either stimulate or challenge the immune system. Some of the environmental factors that affect the immune system are:

Temperature: Temperature can influence the immune system by affecting the activity and survival of immune cells and pathogens. Cold temperatures can reduce the blood flow and mucus production, which can impair the innate immune system and increase the risk of respiratory infections. However, cold temperatures can also stimulate the adaptive immune system by enhancing the production of antibodies and memory cells. Hot temperatures can increase the blood flow and sweating, which can help to flush out toxins and pathogens. However, hot temperatures can also cause dehydration, heat stress, and inflammation, which can weaken the immune system .

Sunlight: Sunlight can affect the immune system by providing ultraviolet (UV) radiation and vitamin D. UV radiation can have both positive and negative effects on the immune system, depending on the dose and duration of exposure.

Low doses of UV radiation can stimulate the immune system by increasing the production of natural killer cells, T cells, and cytokines. However, high doses of UV radiation can suppress the immune system by damaging the DNA and causing skin cancer. Vitamin D can also modulate the immune system by regulating the differentiation and function of immune cells, and enhancing the antimicrobial activity of macrophages and epithelial cells .

Pollution: Pollution can affect the immune system by introducing various chemicals and particles that can trigger or aggravate immune reactions. Air pollution, water pollution, soil pollution, and noise pollution can impair the immune system by causing oxidative stress, inflammation, allergy, asthma, and autoimmune diseases. Pollution can also increase the exposure and susceptibility to infectious agents, such as bacteria, viruses, and fungi .

What are the benefits of having a strong immune system?

Having a strong immune system is beneficial for many reasons, such as:

It helps to prevent and fight off infections and diseases, which can otherwise cause serious complications or even death. A strong immune system can recognize and eliminate harmful invaders, such as bacteria, viruses, parasites, and toxins, before they can cause damage to the body's tissues and organs. A strong immune system can also reduce the severity and duration of symptoms, and speed up the recovery process.

It helps to maintain the balance and harmony of the body's systems and functions, which can otherwise be disrupted by immune disorders. A strong immune system can regulate the immune responses and avoid excessive or inappropriate reactions that can harm the body's own cells and tissues. A strong immune system can also prevent or treat immune disorders, such as allergies, asthma, autoimmune diseases, and immunodeficiencies, which can affect the quality of life and well-being of the affected individuals.

It helps to support the overall health and wellness of the body and mind, which can otherwise be compromised by immune challenges. A strong immune system can protect against oxidative stress and inflammation, which can contribute to aging and chronic diseases. A strong immune system can also enhance the mood and cognition, which can be affected by immune factors, such as cytokines and neurotransmitters. A strong immune system can also improve the response to vaccines and medications, which can increase the effectiveness and safety of the treatments.

How can natural remedies help boost the immune system?

Natural remedies are substances or practices that are derived from nature and have healing or preventive properties.

Natural remedies can help boost the immune system by providing nutrients, antioxidants, anti-inflammatory agents, antimicrobial agents, and immunomodulatory agents that can enhance the function and balance of the immune cells and molecules. Some examples of natural remedies that can help boost the immune system are:

Honey: Honey is a sweet liquid that is produced by bees from the nectar of flowers. Honey has antibacterial, antiviral, antifungal, and anti-inflammatory properties that can help fight infections and reduce inflammation. Honey also contains enzymes, vitamins, minerals, and phytochemicals that can support the immune system. Honey can be consumed raw or added to tea, water, or other beverages. However, honey should not be given to children under one year of age, as it may contain spores of a bacterium that can cause botulism, a serious illness that affects the nervous system .

Garlic: Garlic is a bulbous plant that belongs to the onion family. Garlic has antimicrobial, antiviral, antifungal, and anti-inflammatory properties that can help prevent and treat infections and diseases.

Garlic also contains allicin, a compound that can stimulate the immune system by increasing the activity of natural killer cells, macrophages, and lymphocytes. Garlic can be eaten raw or cooked, or taken as a supplement. However, garlic may interact with some medications, such as blood thinners, and cause bleeding or bruising. Garlic may also cause bad breath, indigestion, or allergic reactions in some people .

Ginger: Ginger is a rhizome or root that is widely used as a spice and a medicine. Ginger has anti-inflammatory, antiviral, antifungal, and antioxidant properties that can help reduce inflammation, fight infections, and protect against oxidative stress. Ginger also contains gingerols, shogaols, and paradols, compounds that can modulate the immune system by regulating the production and release of cytokines, chemokines, and immunoglobulins. Ginger can be consumed fresh, dried, powdered, or as a tea, juice, or oil. However, ginger may cause heartburn, nausea, or diarrhea in some people, and may interact with some medications, such as blood thinners, and increase the risk of bleeding .

Turmeric: Turmeric is a spice that is derived from the root of a plant that belongs to the ginger family. Turmeric has anti-inflammatory, antioxidant, antiviral, and antibacterial properties that can help reduce inflammation, fight infections, and protect against oxidative stress. Turmeric also contains curcumin, a compound that can modulate the immune system by inhibiting the activation of nuclear factor-kappa B (NF-κB), a transcription factor that regulates the expression of genes involved in inflammation, immunity, and cell survival. Turmeric can be added to food, beverages, or supplements. However, turmeric may cause stomach upset, diarrhea, or allergic reactions in some people, and may interact with some medications, such as blood thinners, and make bleeding more likely.

Echinacea: Echinacea is a herb that is native to North America and Europe. Echinacea has immunostimulatory, anti-inflammatory, antiviral, and antibacterial properties that can help enhance the immune system by increasing the number and activity of immune cells, such as natural killer cells, macrophages, and lymphocytes.

Echinacea can also help prevent and treat common colds, flu, and respiratory infections by reducing the severity and duration of symptoms. Echinacea can be taken as a tea, extract, or capsule. However, echinacea may cause allergic reactions, especially in people who are allergic to plants in the same family, such as ragweed, chrysanthemums, marigolds, and daisies. Echinacea may also interact with some medications, such as immunosuppressants, and reduce their effectiveness .

Chapter 1: Nutrition and Immunity

How does nutrition influence the immune system?

Nutrition is one of the most important factors that influence the immune system, as it provides the nutrients and energy that the immune cells need to function properly. Nutrition can affect the immune system in various ways, such as:

Supporting the development and maintenance of the immune cells and molecules: The immune system consists of different types of cells and molecules, such as natural killer cells, macrophages, lymphocytes, antibodies, cytokines, and complement proteins, that work together to protect the body from harmful invaders. These cells and molecules require various nutrients, such as protein, amino acids, fatty acids, vitamins, minerals, and antioxidants, to synthesize, differentiate, proliferate, and activate. A deficiency or excess of these nutrients can impair the immune system by reducing the number and function of the immune cells and molecules, and increasing the risk of infections and diseases .

Modulating the immune responses and balance: The immune system can produce different types of responses, such as innate, adaptive, humoral, cellular, inflammatory, and anti-inflammatory, depending on the nature and severity of the threat. These responses need to be balanced and regulated to avoid excessive or inappropriate reactions that can damage the body's own tissues and organs. Nutrition can modulate the immune system by providing nutrients, such as omega-3 fatty acids, probiotics, prebiotics, and phytochemicals, that can influence the production and release of immune cells and molecules, and enhance or suppress the immune responses and balance .

Protecting against oxidative stress and inflammation: Oxidative stress and inflammation are processes that involve the generation and accumulation of reactive oxygen species (ROS) and pro-inflammatory cytokines, which can cause damage to the cells and tissues, and contribute to aging and chronic diseases. The immune system can protect against oxidative stress and inflammation by producing antioxidants and anti-inflammatory agents, such as glutathione, superoxide dismutase, catalase, and interleukin-10, that can neutralize or reduce the ROS and cytokines. Nutrition can protect against oxidative stress and inflammation by providing nutrients, such as vitamin C, vitamin E, selenium, zinc, and polyphenols, that can act as antioxidants and anti-inflammatory agents, and support the immune system in combating the oxidative stress and inflammation .

What are the essential nutrients for immune health?

The immune system is a complex network of cells, tissues, organs, and molecules that protects the body from harmful invaders, such as bacteria, viruses, parasites, and toxins.

The immune system is essential for our survival, as it helps us fight infections and diseases, and also maintains our overall health and well-being.

To function properly, the immune system needs various nutrients and energy that can be obtained from food, beverages, or supplements. Some of the essential nutrients for immune health are:

Protein: Protein is the building block of the immune cells and molecules, such as antibodies, cytokines, and complement proteins. Protein also helps to repair the damaged tissues and organs after an infection or injury. Protein can be obtained from animal sources, such as meat, eggs, dairy, and fish, or plant sources, such as beans, nuts, seeds, and soy. For adults, the suggested daily amount (RDA) for protein is 0.8 grams per kilogram of body weight.

Amino acids: Amino acids are the components of protein, and some of them have specific roles in the immune system. For example, glutamine is a fuel source for the immune cells, especially the lymphocytes and macrophages. Arginine is involved in the production of nitric oxide, which has antimicrobial and anti-inflammatory effects. Cysteine is a precursor of glutathione, which is a powerful antioxidant that protects the immune cells from oxidative stress. Amino acids can be obtained from protein-rich foods, or from supplements, such as L-glutamine, L-arginine, and N-acetyl cysteine (NAC).

Fatty acids: Fatty acids are the components of fats, and some of them have important functions in the immune system. For example, omega-3 fatty acids, such as eicosapentaenoic acid (EPA) and docosahexaenoic acid (DHA), can modulate the immune system by reducing the production of pro-inflammatory cytokines, and enhancing the activity of natural killer cells and macrophages. Omega-6 fatty acids, such as arachidonic acid (AA) and gamma-linolenic acid (GLA), can also modulate the immune system by regulating the balance between pro-inflammatory and anti-inflammatory responses.

Fatty acids can be obtained from foods, such as fish, flaxseeds, walnuts, and vegetable oils, or from supplements, such as fish oil, flaxseed oil, and evening primrose oil.

Vitamins: Vitamins are organic compounds that are essential for the normal functioning of the immune system. Some of the vitamins that are important for immune health are:

Vitamin A: Vitamin A is involved in the development and maintenance of the mucosal barriers, such as the skin and the respiratory, gastrointestinal, and genitourinary tracts, which are the first line of defense against pathogens. Vitamin A also regulates the differentiation and function of immune cells, such as natural killer cells, macrophages, and lymphocytes. Vitamin A can be obtained from animal sources, such as liver, eggs, dairy, and fish, or from plant sources, such as carrots, sweet potatoes, spinach, and mangoes. The RDA for vitamin A is 900 micrograms for men and 700 micrograms for women per day.

Vitamin C: Vitamin C is a potent antioxidant that can protect the immune cells from oxidative stress and enhance their activity. Vitamin C also stimulates the production and function of immune cells and molecules, such as natural killer cells, macrophages, lymphocytes, antibodies, and cytokines. Vitamin C can also help to prevent and treat infections and diseases, such as colds, flu, and pneumonia, by reducing the severity and duration of symptoms. Vitamin C can be obtained from fruits and vegetables, such as citrus fruits, berries, kiwi, broccoli, and peppers. The RDA for vitamin C is 90 milligrams for men and 75 milligrams for women per day.

Vitamin D: Vitamin D is a hormone that can modulate the immune system by regulating the expression of genes involved in immunity, inflammation, and cell survival. Vitamin D also enhances the antimicrobial activity of macrophages and epithelial cells, and inhibits the proliferation and activation of immune cells, such as T cells and B cells. Vitamin D can also help to prevent and treat immune disorders, such as autoimmune diseases, allergies, and asthma, by maintaining the immune tolerance and balance. Vitamin D can be obtained from exposure to sunlight, or from foods, such as fatty fish, egg yolks, mushrooms, and fortified foods, or from supplements. The RDA for vitamin D is 15 micrograms for adults under 70 years of age and 20 micrograms for adults over 70 years of age per day.

Vitamin E: Vitamin E is another antioxidant that can protect the immune cells from oxidative stress and enhance their function. Vitamin E also modulates the immune system by influencing the production and release of cytokines, chemokines, and immunoglobulins. Vitamin E can also help to prevent and treat infections and diseases, such as herpes, hepatitis, and HIV, by inhibiting the replication and entry of viruses. Vitamin E can be obtained from foods, such as nuts, seeds, vegetable oils, and wheat germ. The RDA for vitamin E is 15 milligrams for adults per day.

Vitamin B6: Vitamin B6 is involved in the metabolism of amino acids, which are the components of protein and the immune cells and molecules. Vitamin B6 also supports the production and function of immune cells and molecules, such as natural killer cells, macrophages, lymphocytes, antibodies, and cytokines. Vitamin B6 can also help to prevent and treat infections and diseases, such as tuberculosis, malaria, and HIV, by enhancing the immune responses and balance. Vitamin B6 can be obtained from foods, such as meat, poultry, fish, eggs, dairy, and bananas. The RDA for vitamin B6 is 1.3 milligrams for adults under 50 years of age and 1.7 milligrams for men and 1.5 milligrams for women over 50 years of age per day.

Vitamin B12: Vitamin B12 is involved in the synthesis of DNA and RNA, which are the genetic material of the immune cells and molecules. Vitamin B12 also supports the production and function of immune cells and molecules, such as natural killer cells, macrophages, lymphocytes, antibodies, and cytokines. Vitamin B12 can also help to prevent and treat infections and diseases, such as anemia, pernicious anemia, and HIV, by maintaining the red blood cell and nerve function. Vitamin B12 can be obtained from animal sources, such as meat, eggs, dairy, and fish, or from supplements. The RDA for vitamin B12 is 2.4 micrograms for adults per day.

Minerals: Minerals are inorganic elements that are essential for the normal functioning of the immune system. Some of the minerals that are important for immune health are:

Zinc: Zinc is a cofactor for many enzymes that are involved in the immune system, such as superoxide dismutase, catalase, and glutathione peroxidase, which are antioxidants that protect the immune cells from oxidative stress. Zinc also supports the production and function of immune cells and molecules, such as natural killer cells, macrophages, lymphocytes, antibodies, and cytokines. Zinc can also help to prevent and treat infections and diseases, such as colds, flu, diarrhea, and pneumonia, by enhancing the immune responses and balance. Zinc can be obtained from foods, such as meat, seafood, nuts, seeds, and whole grains, or from supplements. The RDA for zinc is 11 milligrams for men and 8 milligrams for women per day.

Selenium: Selenium is another cofactor for many enzymes that are involved in the immune system, such as glutathione peroxidase, thioredoxin reductase, and selenoprotein P, which are antioxidants that protect the immune cells from oxidative stress. Selenium also modulates the immune system by influencing the production and release of cytokines, chemokines, and immunoglobulins. Selenium can also help to prevent and treat infections and diseases, such as viral infections, hepatitis, and HIV, by inhibiting the replication and entry of viruses. Selenium can be obtained from foods, such as Brazil nuts, fish, meat, eggs, and mushrooms, or from supplements. Adults should consume 55 micrograms of selenium daily.

Iron: Iron is a component of hemoglobin, which is a protein that carries oxygen to the immune cells and tissues. Iron also supports the production and function of immune cells and molecules, such as natural killer cells, macrophages, lymphocytes, antibodies, and cytokines. Iron can also help to prevent and treat infections and diseases, such as anemia, malaria, and tuberculosis, by enhancing the immune responses and balance. Iron can be obtained from foods, such as meat, poultry, fish, eggs, beans, and spinach, or from supplements.

The RDA for iron is 8 milligrams for men and 18 milligrams for women per day.

Copper: Copper is another component of many enzymes that are involved in the immune system, such as superoxide dismutase, ceruloplasmin, and lysyl oxidase, which are antioxidants that protect the immune cells from oxidative stress. Copper also supports the production and function of immune cells and molecules, such as natural killer cells, macrophages, lymphocytes, antibodies, and cytok

What are the best foods to eat to boost the immune system?

Some of the best foods to eat to boost the immune system are:

Citrus fruits: Citrus fruits, such as oranges, grapefruits, lemons, and limes, are rich in vitamin C, which is a potent antioxidant that can protect the immune cells from oxidative stress and enhance their activity.

Vitamin C also stimulates the production and function of immune cells and molecules, such as natural killer cells, macrophages, lymphocytes, antibodies, and cytokines. Vitamin C can also help to prevent and treat infections and diseases, such as colds, flu, and pneumonia, by reducing the severity and duration of symptoms. Citrus fruits can be eaten fresh, juiced, or added to salads, smoothies, or desserts.

Berries: Berries, such as blueberries, strawberries, raspberries, and cranberries, are also rich in vitamin C, as well as other antioxidants, such as anthocyanins, flavonoids, and phenolic acids, that can protect the immune cells from oxidative stress and enhance their function. Berries also contain phytochemicals, such as ellagic acid, resveratrol, and quercetin, that can modulate the immune system by influencing the production and release of cytokines, chemokines, and immunoglobulins. Berries can also help to prevent and treat infections and diseases, such as urinary tract infections, by inhibiting the adhesion and growth of bacteria. Berries can be eaten fresh, frozen, dried, or added to yogurt, oatmeal, or baked goods.

Yogurt: Yogurt is a fermented dairy product that contains probiotics, which are beneficial bacteria that can colonize the gut and support the immune system. Probiotics can modulate the immune system by enhancing the activity of natural killer cells, macrophages, and lymphocytes, and by producing antimicrobial substances, such as lactic acid, hydrogen peroxide, and bacteriocins. Probiotics can also help to prevent and treat infections and diseases, such as diarrhea, irritable bowel syndrome, and inflammatory bowel disease, by maintaining the gut barrier and balance. Yogurt can be eaten plain, flavored, or mixed with fruits, nuts, seeds, or granola.

Garlic: Garlic is a bulbous plant that belongs to the onion family. Garlic has antimicrobial, antiviral, antifungal, and anti-inflammatory properties that can help prevent and treat infections and diseases. Garlic also contains allicin, a compound that can stimulate the immune system by increasing the activity of natural killer cells, macrophages, and lymphocytes. Garlic can be eaten raw or cooked, or taken as a supplement.

However, garlic may interact with some medications, such as blood thinners, and cause bleeding or bruising. Garlic may also cause bad breath, indigestion, or allergic reactions in some people.

Ginger: Ginger is a rhizome or root that is widely used as a spice and a medicine. Ginger has anti-inflammatory, antiviral, antifungal, and antioxidant properties that can help reduce inflammation, fight infections, and protect against oxidative stress. Ginger also contains gingerols, shogaols, and paradols, compounds that can modulate the immune system by regulating the production and release of cytokines, chemokines, and immunoglobulins. Ginger can be consumed fresh, dried, powdered, or as a tea, juice, or oil. However, ginger may cause heartburn, nausea, or diarrhea in some people, and may interact with some medications, such as blood thinners, and increase the risk of bleeding.

What are the foods to avoid or limit to prevent immune suppression?

Some of the foods to avoid or limit to prevent immune suppression are:

Processed foods: Processed foods are foods that have been altered from their natural state, and usually contain additives, preservatives, artificial colors, flavors, and sweeteners. Processed foods can impair the immune system by causing nutrient deficiencies, dysbiosis, obesity, and metabolic disorders. Processed foods can also increase the production of pro-inflammatory cytokines, and reduce the activity of natural killer cells and macrophages. Processed foods include fast foods, junk foods, canned foods, frozen foods, and ready meals.

Refined sugars: Refined sugars are sugars that have been extracted and purified from their natural sources, such as sugarcane, beet, or corn. Refined sugars can impair the immune system by causing nutrient deficiencies, dysbiosis, obesity, and metabolic disorders. Refined sugars can also increase the production of pro-inflammatory cytokines, and reduce the activity of natural killer cells and lymphocytes.

Refined sugars include table sugar, high-fructose corn syrup, glucose, fructose, and sucrose.

Saturated fats: Saturated fats are fats that are solid at room temperature, and usually come from animal sources, such as meat, dairy, and eggs. Saturated fats can impair the immune system by causing nutrient deficiencies, dysbiosis, obesity, and metabolic disorders. Saturated fats can also increase the production of pro-inflammatory cytokines, and reduce the activity of natural killer cells and macrophages. Saturated fats include butter, cheese, cream, lard, and bacon.

Alcohol: Alcohol is a psychoactive substance that can affect the brain and the nervous system. Alcohol can impair the immune system by causing nutrient deficiencies, dysbiosis, dehydration, and liver damage. Alcohol can also increase the production of pro-inflammatory cytokines, and reduce the activity of natural killer cells, macrophages, and lymphocytes. Alcohol can also increase the exposure and susceptibility to infectious agents, such as bacteria, viruses, and fungi. Alcohol includes beer, wine, liquor, and spirits.

Chapter 2: Herbs and Supplements for Immunity

How do herbs and supplements support the immune system?

Herbs and supplements are substances or products that are derived from plants, animals, minerals, or synthetic sources, and have medicinal or health-promoting properties. Herbs and supplements can support the immune system by providing nutrients, antioxidants, anti-inflammatory agents, antimicrobial agents, and immunomodulatory agents that can enhance the function and balance of the immune cells and molecules. Some examples of herbs and supplements that can support the immune system are:

Echinacea: Echinacea is a herb that is native to North America and Europe.

Echinacea has immunostimulatory, anti-inflammatory, antiviral, and antibacterial properties that can help enhance the immune system by increasing the number and activity of immune cells, such as natural killer cells, macrophages, and lymphocytes. Echinacea can also help prevent and treat common colds, flu, and respiratory infections by reducing the severity and duration of symptoms. Echinacea can be taken as a tea, extract, or capsule. However, echinacea may cause allergic reactions, especially in people who are allergic to plants in the same family, such as ragweed, chrysanthemums, marigolds, and daisies. Echinacea may also interact with some medications, such as immunosuppressants, and reduce their effectiveness .

Ginseng: Ginseng is a root that is widely used as a tonic and an adaptogen. Ginseng has immunomodulatory, anti-inflammatory, antioxidant, and antiviral properties that can help modulate the immune system by regulating the production and release of cytokines, chemokines, and immunoglobulins. Ginseng can also help to prevent and treat infections and diseases, such as herpes, hepatitis, and HIV, by inhibiting the replication and entry of viruses. Ginseng can be consumed as a tea, powder, or capsule. However, ginseng may cause side effects, such as insomnia, headache, nausea, or diarrhea, and may interact with some medications, such as blood thinners, and increase the risk of bleeding .

Turmeric: Turmeric is a spice that is derived from the root of a plant that belongs to the ginger family. Turmeric has anti-inflammatory, antioxidant, antiviral, and antibacterial properties that can help reduce inflammation, fight infections, and protect against oxidative stress. Turmeric also contains curcumin, a compound that can modulate the immune system by inhibiting the activation of nuclear factor-kappa B (NF-κB), a transcription factor that regulates the expression of genes involved in inflammation, immunity, and cell survival. Turmeric can be added to food, beverages, or supplements. However, turmeric may cause stomach upset, diarrhea, or allergic reactions in some people, and may interact with some medications, such as blood thinners, and increase the risk of bleeding .

Vitamin C: Vitamin C is a potent antioxidant that can protect the immune cells from oxidative stress and enhance their activity. Vitamin C also stimulates the production and function of immune cells and molecules, such as natural killer cells, macrophages, lymphocytes, antibodies, and cytokines. Vitamin C can also help to prevent and treat infections and diseases, such as colds, flu, and pneumonia, by reducing the severity and duration of symptoms. Vitamin C can be obtained from fruits and vegetables, such as citrus fruits, berries, kiwi, broccoli, and peppers, or from supplements. The RDA for vitamin C is 90 milligrams for men and 75 milligrams for women per day .

Zinc: Zinc is a cofactor for many enzymes that are involved in the immune system, such as superoxide dismutase, catalase, and glutathione peroxidase, which are antioxidants that protect the immune cells from oxidative stress. Zinc also supports the production and function of immune cells and molecules, such as natural killer cells, macrophages, lymphocytes, antibodies, and cytokines.

Zinc can also help to prevent and treat infections and diseases, such as colds, flu, diarrhea, and pneumonia, by enhancing the immune responses and balance. Zinc can be obtained from foods, such as meat, seafood, nuts, seeds, and whole grains, or from supplements. The RDA for zinc is 11 milligrams for men and 8 milligrams for women per day .

What are the most effective herbs and supplements for immune health?

There are many herbs and supplements that can support the immune system, but some of them may be more effective than others, depending on the individual's needs, preferences, and conditions. However, based on the current scientific evidence, some of the most effective herbs and supplements for immune health are:

Echinacea: Echinacea is a herb that is native to North America and Europe. Echinacea has immunostimulatory, anti-inflammatory, antiviral, and antibacterial properties that can help enhance the immune system by increasing the number and activity of immune cells, such as natural killer cells, macrophages, and lymphocytes. Echinacea can also help prevent and treat common colds, flu, and respiratory infections by reducing the severity and duration of symptoms. Echinacea can be taken as a tea, extract, or capsule. However, echinacea may cause allergic reactions, especially in people who are allergic to plants in the similar family, including chrysan and ragweed. Echinacea may also interact with some medications, such as immunosuppressants, and reduce their effectiveness .

Ginseng: Ginseng is a root that is widely used as a tonic and an adaptogen. Ginseng has immunomodulatory, anti-inflammatory, antioxidant, and antiviral properties that can help modulate the immune system by regulating the production and release of cytokines, chemokines, and immunoglobulins. Ginseng can also help to prevent and treat infections and diseases, such as herpes, hepatitis, and HIV, by inhibiting the replication and entry of viruses. Ginseng can be consumed as a tea, powder, or capsule.

However, ginseng may cause side effects, such as insomnia, headache, nausea, or diarrhea, and may interact with some medications, such as blood thinners, and increase the risk of bleeding .

Turmeric: Turmeric is a spice that is derived from the root of a plant that belongs to the ginger family. Turmeric has anti-inflammatory, antioxidant, antiviral, and antibacterial properties that can help reduce inflammation, fight infections, and protect against oxidative stress. Turmeric also contains curcumin, a compound that can modulate the immune system by inhibiting the activation of nuclear factor-kappa B (NF-κB), a transcription factor that regulates the expression of genes involved in inflammation, immunity, and cell survival. Turmeric can be added to food, beverages, or supplements. However, turmeric may cause stomach upset, diarrhea, or allergic reactions in some people, and may interact with some medications, such as blood thinners, and increase the risk of bleeding .

Vitamin C: Vitamin C is a potent antioxidant that can protect the immune cells from oxidative stress and enhance their activity.

Vitamin C also stimulates the production and function of immune cells and molecules, such as natural killer cells, macrophages, lymphocytes, antibodies, and cytokines. Vitamin C can also help to prevent and treat infections and diseases, such as colds, flu, and pneumonia, by reducing the severity and duration of symptoms. Vitamin C can be obtained from fruits and vegetables, such as citrus fruits, berries, kiwi, broccoli, and peppers, or from supplements. The RDA for vitamin C is 90 milligrams for men and 75 milligrams for women per day .

Zinc: Zinc is a cofactor for many enzymes that are involved in the immune system, such as superoxide dismutase, catalase, and glutathione peroxidase, which are antioxidants that protect the immune cells from oxidative stress. Zinc also supports the production and function of immune cells and molecules, such as natural killer cells, macrophages, lymphocytes, antibodies, and cytokines. Zinc can also help to prevent and treat infections and diseases, such as colds, flu, diarrhea, and pneumonia, by enhancing the immune responses and balance.

Zinc can be obtained from foods, such as meat, seafood, nuts, seeds, and whole grains, or from supplements. The RDA for zinc is 11 milligrams for men and 8 milligrams for women per day .

These are some of the most effective herbs and supplements for immune health, but they are not the only ones. There are many other herbs and supplements that can also support the immune system, such as garlic, ginger, vitamin D, selenium, iron, copper, magnesium, and more. However, before taking any herbs or supplements, it is advisable to consult with a doctor or a health professional, as they may have side effects or interactions with other medications or conditions. It is also important to follow the recommended dosage and duration, and to choose high-quality products from reputable sources. Herbs and supplements can complement, but not replace, a healthy diet, lifestyle, and medical care for immune health.

How to use herbs and supplements safely and effectively?

Herbs and supplements are substances or products that can support the immune system by providing various benefits, such as nutrients, antioxidants, anti-inflammatory agents, antimicrobial agents, and immunomodulatory agents. However, herbs and supplements are not regulated by the Food and Drug Administration (FDA), and they may have side effects or interactions with other medications or conditions. Therefore, it is important to use herbs and supplements safely and effectively, by following these tips:

Consult with a doctor or a health professional before taking any herbs or supplements: This is especially important if you have any medical conditions, allergies, or are pregnant or breastfeeding. A doctor or a health professional can help you determine the appropriate type, dosage, and duration of the herbs or supplements, and monitor your progress and reactions.

They can also advise you on any potential side effects or interactions with other medications or supplements that you are taking, and how to avoid or manage them.

Choose high-quality products from reputable sources: Not all herbs and supplements are created equal, and some of them may contain contaminants, additives, or incorrect ingredients or amounts. Therefore, it is important to choose high-quality products from reputable sources, such as certified organic, non-GMO, or third-party tested. You can also check the labels and the websites of the products for information on the ingredients, sources, manufacturing, and testing methods, and look for seals of approval from independent organizations, such as the U.S. Pharmacopeia (USP), the National Sanitation Foundation (NSF), or the ConsumerLab.com.

Follow the recommended dosage and duration: Taking too much or too little of the herbs or supplements, or taking them for too long or too short, can affect their effectiveness and safety. Therefore, it is important to follow the recommended dosage and duration of the herbs or supplements, as suggested by the doctor or the health professional, or by the product label or the website. You can also use a measuring spoon, cup, or scale to ensure the accurate amount of the herbs or supplements, and keep a record of when and how much you take them.

Be aware of the possible side effects or interactions: Even though herbs and supplements are natural, they can still cause side effects or interactions with other medications or supplements, or with certain foods or beverages. Some of the common side effects or interactions of herbs and supplements are:

Allergic reactions: Some people may be allergic to certain herbs or supplements, or to their components, such as pollen, latex, or gluten. Allergic reactions can range from mild to severe, and can include symptoms such as rash, itching, swelling, hives, difficulty breathing, or anaphylaxis. If you experience any signs of an allergic reaction, stop taking the herbs or supplements immediately, and seek medical attention.

Bleeding or bruising: Some herbs or supplements, such as garlic, ginger, ginseng, turmeric, vitamin E, and omega-3 fatty acids, can thin the blood and increase the risk of bleeding or bruising, especially if taken with blood thinners, such as warfarin, aspirin, or ibuprofen. If you are taking any blood thinners, or have any bleeding disorders, consult with your doctor before taking these herbs or supplements, and monitor your blood clotting and platelet levels regularly.

Digestive issues: Some herbs or supplements, such as echinacea, zinc, iron, copper, magnesium, and probiotics, can cause digestive issues, such as nausea, vomiting, diarrhea, constipation, or abdominal pain, especially if taken on an empty stomach, or in large doses. If you experience any digestive issues, try taking the herbs or supplements with food, or reduce the dose, or switch to a different form, such as liquid, capsule, or powder. You can also drink plenty of water, and eat foods that are rich in fiber, to ease the digestion and absorption of the herbs or supplements.

Liver damage: Some herbs or supplements, such as kava, comfrey, chaparral, and vitamin A, can cause liver damage, especially if taken in high doses, or for a long time, or with alcohol, or with other medications that affect the liver, such as acetaminophen, statins, or antibiotics. Liver damage can cause symptoms such as jaundice, dark urine, pale stools, fatigue, loss of appetite, or abdominal pain. If you have any liver problems, or are taking any medications that affect the liver, consult with your doctor before taking these herbs or supplements, and monitor your liver function tests regularly.

Hormonal changes: Some herbs or supplements, such as ginseng, licorice, soy, black cohosh, and vitamin D, can affect the hormonal balance, especially if taken in high doses, or for a long time, or with other hormones, such as birth control pills, hormone replacement therapy, or thyroid medications. Hormonal changes can cause symptoms such as acne, hair loss, weight gain, mood swings, irregular periods, or breast tenderness. If you have any hormonal problems, or are taking any hormones, consult with your doctor before taking these herbs or supplements, and monitor your hormone levels regularly.

These are some of the tips on how to use herbs and supplements safely and effectively, but they are not the only ones. There are many other factors that can affect the effectiveness and safety of herbs and supplements, such as the individual's age, weight, health status, and genetic makeup. Therefore, it is important to do your own research, and consult with a doctor or a health professional, before taking any herbs or supplements, and to follow their instructions and recommendations. Herbs and supplements can complement, but not replace, a healthy diet, lifestyle, and medical care for immune health.

What are the possible interactions and side effects of herbs and supplements?

Herbs and supplements are natural products that can have various effects on the body. Some of them may interact with medicines, either by enhancing or reducing their effects, or by causing unwanted side effects.

Therefore, it is important to be aware of the possible interactions and side effects of herbs and supplements, especially if you are taking any prescription or over-the-counter medicines.

Here are some examples of herbs and supplements that can interact with medicines:

St. John's wort is an herb that is often used for depression, anxiety, and insomnia. However, it can interact with many types of drugs, such as antidepressants, birth control pills, blood thinners, HIV drugs, and others. In most cases, it speeds up the breakdown of these drugs in the body, leading to lower levels and reduced effectiveness. It can also cause serious side effects, such as serotonin syndrome, when taken with certain antidepressants.

Garlic is a common ingredient in many cuisines and has been used for various health benefits, such as lowering blood pressure and cholesterol, and preventing infections. However, garlic can also thin the blood, similar to aspirin, and increase the risk of bleeding. This can be a problem for people who take blood thinners, such as warfarin, or who have surgery or dental procedures.

Green tea is a popular beverage that contains antioxidants and other compounds that may have anti-inflammatory, anti-cancer, and weight-loss effects. However, green tea can also interact with some decongestants, such as pseudoephedrine, and cause a rise in blood pressure and heart rate. This can be dangerous for people who have heart or blood vessel problems[2].

Goldenseal is an herb that is often used for digestive issues, infections, and skin problems. However, it can also affect the metabolism of some drugs, such as cyclosporine, digoxin, and warfarin, and alter their levels in the body. This can lead to either toxicity or reduced effectiveness of these drugs. Goldenseal has a high risk of interaction with many medicines and should be used with caution.

These are just some of the examples of herbs and supplements that can interact with medicines. There are many others that may have similar or different effects. Therefore, it is advisable to consult your health care provider before taking any herbs or supplements, especially if you are taking any medicines or have any medical conditions. You should also inform your health care provider about all the herbs and supplements you are taking, and report any side effects or changes in your health. By doing so, you can avoid potential interactions and side effects, and use herbs and supplements safely and effectively.

Chapter 3: Lifestyle and Immunity

How does lifestyle affect the immune system?

Lifestyle is a term that encompasses many aspects of our daily habits, choices, and behaviors. Lifestyle can affect the immune system in various ways, either positively or negatively. The body's defense against pathogenic invaders like bacteria, viruses, fungi, and parasites is provided by the immune system, which is an intricate network of cells, tissues, and organs. The immune system also helps to regulate inflammation, which is a normal response to injury or infection, but can become chronic and harmful if not controlled.

Some of the lifestyle factors that can influence the immune system are:

Diet: Diet plays a crucial role in providing the nutrients and antioxidants that the immune system needs to function properly. A balanced diet that includes a variety of fruits, vegetables, whole grains, lean proteins, healthy fats, and probiotics can help to support the immune system and prevent deficiencies. Some of the nutrients that are especially important for the immune system are vitamin C, vitamin D, zinc, selenium, iron, and omega-3 fatty acids. On the other hand, a diet that is high in processed foods, added sugars, saturated fats, and alcohol can impair the immune system and increase inflammation.

Exercise: Exercise can have both positive and negative effects on the immune system, depending on the type, intensity, duration, and frequency of the physical activity. Moderate exercise, such as brisk walking, cycling, or swimming, can enhance the immune system by improving blood circulation, reducing stress, and lowering the risk of chronic diseases, such as obesity, diabetes, and cardiovascular disease. However, excessive or strenuous exercise, such as marathon running, can suppress the immune system and increase the risk of infections, especially in the upper respiratory tract. Therefore, it is important to find a balance between rest and exercise, and to listen to your body's signals.

Sleep: Sleep is essential for the immune system, as it allows the body to repair and regenerate its cells and tissues, and to produce and release immune molecules, such as cytokines, antibodies, and natural killer cells. Lack of sleep or poor quality sleep can impair the immune system and increase the susceptibility to infections, inflammation, and chronic diseases. The optimal amount of sleep may vary from person to person, but generally, adults need about 7 to 9 hours of sleep per night, while children and adolescents need more.

Smoking: Smoking is one of the most harmful lifestyle factors for the immune system, as it exposes the body to thousands of toxic chemicals that can damage the cells and tissues of the immune system, and interfere with its normal functioning. Smoking can increase the risk of infections, such as pneumonia, tuberculosis, and influenza, and chronic diseases, such as cancer, chronic obstructive pulmonary disease, and cardiovascular disease. Quitting smoking can improve the immune system and reduce the risk of these diseases.

Stress: Stress is a natural and inevitable part of life, but when it becomes chronic or overwhelming, it can have negative effects on the immune system. Stress can activate the sympathetic nervous system and the hypothalamic-pituitary-adrenal axis, which release hormones, such as adrenaline, cortisol, and norepinephrine, that can suppress the immune system and increase inflammation. Chronic stress can also affect the behavior and mood of the person, leading to unhealthy coping strategies, such as overeating, smoking, drinking, or drug abuse, which can further impair the immune system. Therefore, it is important to manage stress in healthy ways, such as meditation, yoga, breathing exercises, hobbies, social support, and counseling.

Age: Age is another factor that can affect the immune system, as it undergoes changes throughout the lifespan. The immune system is immature in infants and children, making them more vulnerable to infections and allergies, but also more responsive to vaccinations and immune therapies. The immune system reaches its peak in young adulthood, and then gradually declines with age, a process known as immunosenescence[12]. This can result in reduced immune function, increased inflammation, and increased risk of infections, autoimmune diseases, and cancer in older adults[12]. However, some of the effects of aging on the immune system can be modulated by lifestyle factors, such as diet, exercise, sleep, and stress.

Medical conditions: Some medical conditions can also affect the immune system, either by causing it to be overactive or underactive. For example, autoimmune diseases, such as rheumatoid arthritis, lupus, and type 1 diabetes, are characterized by an abnormal immune response that attacks the body's own tissues, causing inflammation and damage. On the other hand, immunodeficiency diseases, such as HIV/AIDS, primary immunodeficiency, and cancer, are characterized by a weakened or absent immune response that fails to protect the body from infections and tumors. These conditions require medical attention and treatment, which may include immunosuppressive drugs, immunomodulators, or immunotherapy.

As you can see, lifestyle can have a significant impact on the immune system, and therefore, on the overall health and well-being of the person. By adopting a healthy lifestyle that includes a balanced diet, moderate exercise, adequate sleep, smoking cessation, stress management, and regular check-ups, you can help to strengthen your immune system and prevent or treat many diseases. Remember, your immune system is your best ally in fighting off germs and staying healthy.

What are the best practices to enhance the immune system?

The immune system is the body's defense mechanism against harmful invaders, such as bacteria, viruses, fungi, and parasites. A strong immune system can help prevent or fight off infections and diseases, while a weak immune system can make you more susceptible to illness.

There are many factors that can affect the immune system, such as age, genetics, medical conditions, and environmental exposures. However, there are also some lifestyle choices that can enhance the immune system and improve your overall health and well-being.

Get enough sleep: Sleep is essential for the immune system, as it allows the body to repair and regenerate its cells and tissues, and to produce and release immune molecules, such as cytokines, antibodies, and natural killer cells. Lack of sleep or poor quality sleep can impair the immune system and increase the susceptibility to infections, inflammation, and chronic diseases. Adults should aim to get 7 or more hours of sleep per night, while teens need 8–10 hours and younger children and infants up to 14 hours.

Eat a balanced diet: Diet plays a crucial role in providing the nutrients and antioxidants that the immune system needs to function properly. A balanced diet that includes a variety of fruits, vegetables, nuts, seeds, and legumes can help to support the immune system and prevent deficiencies. Some of the nutrients that are especially important for the immune system are vitamin C, vitamin D, zinc, selenium, iron, and omega-3 fatty acids[12]. On the other hand, a diet that is high in processed foods, added sugars, saturated fats, and alcohol can impair the immune system and increase inflammation[12].

Exercise moderately: Exercise can have both positive and negative effects on the immune system, depending on the type, intensity, duration, and frequency of the physical activity. Moderate exercise, such as brisk walking, cycling, or swimming, can enhance the immune system by improving blood circulation, reducing stress, and lowering the risk of chronic diseases, such as obesity, diabetes, and cardiovascular disease. However, excessive or strenuous exercise, such as marathon running, can suppress the immune system and increase the risk of infections, especially in the upper respiratory tract. Therefore, it is important to find a balance between rest and exercise, and to listen to your body's signals.

Manage stress: Stress is a natural and inevitable part of life, but when it becomes chronic or overwhelming, it can have negative effects on the immune system. Stress can activate the sympathetic nervous system and the hypothalamic-pituitary-adrenal axis, which release hormones, such as adrenaline, cortisol, and norepinephrine, that can suppress the immune system and increase inflammation. Chronic stress can also affect the behavior and mood of the person, leading to unhealthy coping strategies, such as overeating, smoking, drinking, or drug abuse, which can further impair the immune system. Therefore, it is important to manage stress in healthy ways, such as meditation, yoga, breathing exercises, hobbies, social support, and counseling.

Quit smoking: Smoking is one of the most harmful lifestyle factors for the immune system, as it exposes the body to thousands of toxic chemicals that can damage the cells and tissues of the immune system, and interfere with its normal functioning. Smoking can increase the risk of infections, such as pneumonia, tuberculosis, and influenza, and chronic diseases, such as cancer, chronic obstructive pulmonary disease, and cardiovascular disease. Quitting smoking can improve the immune system and reduce the risk of these diseases.

Get vaccinated: Vaccines are one of the most effective ways to prevent infectious diseases and boost the immune system. Vaccines work by exposing the body to a weakened or inactive form of a pathogen, which stimulates the immune system to produce antibodies and memory cells that can recognize and fight off the same or similar pathogens in the future. Vaccines can protect you from diseases such as measles, mumps, rubella, polio, tetanus, diphtheria, pertussis, hepatitis, meningitis, influenza, and COVID-19. It is important to follow the recommended vaccination schedule and get booster shots when needed.

These are some of the best practices to enhance the immune system and improve your health. However, keep in mind that these are not specific to COVID-19, and that no supplement, diet, or lifestyle modification can protect you from developing COVID-19. The best way to prevent COVID-19 is to follow the public health guidelines, such as wearing a mask, practicing physical distancing, washing your hands frequently, and avoiding large gatherings.

How to manage stress, sleep, exercise, and hygiene for immune health?

The intricate network of cells, tissues, and organs that makes up the immune system shields the body against dangerous invaders such as bacteria, viruses, fungi, and parasites. As a natural reaction to damage or infection, inflammation is another function of the immune system.

However, when the immune system is not functioning properly, it can cause problems such as allergies, autoimmune diseases, chronic infections, and cancer.

One of the factors that can affect the immune system is the lifestyle of the individual. Stress, sleep, exercise, and hygiene are some of the aspects of lifestyle that can have a positive or negative impact on the immune system. Here are some tips on how to manage these factors for optimal immune health:

Stress: Stress is a natural and unavoidable part of life, but too much stress can weaken the immune system and make it more susceptible to infections and diseases. Stress can also trigger or worsen inflammation, which can damage the body's tissues and organs. Therefore, it is important to find healthy ways to cope with stress, such as relaxation techniques, meditation, yoga, breathing exercises, hobbies, social support, counseling, or therapy. Avoiding or limiting the sources of stress, such as work, family, or financial issues, can also help to reduce the stress level.

Sleep: Sleep is essential for the immune system, as it allows the body to rest, repair, and regenerate. During sleep, the immune system produces and releases various molecules that help to fight infections and inflammation, such as cytokines, antibodies, and natural killer cells. Lack of sleep or poor quality sleep can impair the immune system and raise the possibility of illnesses and infections. Therefore, it is recommended to get at least seven to eight hours of sleep per night, and to follow good sleep hygiene practices, such as having a regular sleep schedule, avoiding caffeine, alcohol, nicotine, and heavy meals before bedtime, keeping the bedroom dark, quiet, and comfortable, and avoiding the use of electronic devices before or during sleep.

Exercise: Exercise is beneficial for the immune system, as it helps to improve blood circulation, oxygen delivery, and lymphatic drainage, which are all important for the immune system's function. Exercise also helps to reduce stress, improve mood, and enhance sleep quality, which can also boost the immune system. However, too much or too intense exercise can have the opposite effect, as it can cause physical and mental stress, inflammation, and tissue damage, which can impair the immune system and increase the risk of infections and diseases. Therefore, it is advised to follow a moderate and balanced exercise routine, which includes aerobic, strength, and flexibility exercises, and to rest and recover adequately between workouts.

Hygiene: Hygiene is another factor that can influence the immune system, as it helps to prevent the exposure and transmission of harmful germs that can cause infections and diseases. Hygiene practices include washing the hands frequently and thoroughly with soap and water, especially before and after eating, after using the bathroom, after coughing, sneezing, or blowing the nose, and after touching potentially contaminated surfaces or objects. Hygiene also involves covering the mouth and nose with a tissue or elbow when coughing or sneezing, and disposing of the tissue properly. Hygiene also includes keeping the body, hair, nails, teeth, and clothes clean, and avoiding sharing personal items such as towels, toothbrushes, razors, or utensils.

Hygiene also means staying home and seeking medical attention when sick, and following the recommended vaccination schedule to prevent certain diseases.

How to avoid or reduce exposure to toxins and pathogens that weaken the immune system.

The body is shielded from dangerous invaders like bacteria, viruses, fungi, and parasites by the intricate network of cells, tissues, and organs that make up the immune system. The immune system also helps to regulate inflammation, which is a normal response to injury or infection. However, the immune system can also be affected by external factors, such as toxins and pathogens, that can weaken its function and increase the risk of infections and diseases.

Toxins are substances that can cause damage to the cells and tissues of the body, and interfere with the normal functioning of the organs and systems. Toxins can come from various sources, such as air pollution, water contamination, food additives, pesticides, drugs, alcohol, tobacco, cosmetics, household products, and industrial waste. Toxins can also be produced by the body itself, as a result of metabolic processes or infections.

Pathogens are microorganisms that can cause infections and diseases in the body, such as bacteria, viruses, fungi, and parasites. Pathogens can enter the body through various routes, such as inhalation, ingestion, skin contact, sexual contact, or insect bites. Pathogens can also be transmitted from person to person, or from animals to humans.

To avoid or reduce exposure to toxins and pathogens that weaken the immune system, here are some tips to follow:

Toxins: To reduce the exposure to toxins, it is advisable to avoid or limit the use of substances that can harm the body, such as drugs, alcohol, tobacco, and caffeine. It is also important to choose organic, fresh, and unprocessed foods, and to wash them thoroughly before consumption. It is also recommended to drink filtered or purified water, and to avoid plastic bottles or containers that can leach chemicals into the water. It is also beneficial to use natural or eco-friendly products for personal care, cleaning, and gardening, and to avoid synthetic fragrances, dyes, and preservatives. It is also essential to avoid or minimize the exposure to air pollution, by using air purifiers, masks, or filters, and by avoiding smoking or secondhand smoke. It is also helpful to detoxify the body regularly, by eating foods that support the liver, kidneys, and colon, such as cruciferous vegetables, garlic, onion, turmeric, ginger, lemon, apple, beetroot, and flaxseed. It is also advisable to exercise, sweat, and hydrate, to help the body eliminate toxins through the skin, lungs, and urine.

Pathogens: To avoid or reduce the exposure to pathogens, it is crucial to practice good hygiene, such as washing the hands frequently and thoroughly with soap and water, especially before and after eating, after using the bathroom, after coughing, sneezing, or blowing the nose, and after touching potentially contaminated surfaces or objects. It is also important to cover the mouth and nose with a tissue or elbow when coughing or sneezing, and to dispose of the tissue properly. It is also necessary to keep the body, hair, nails, teeth, and clothes clean, and to avoid sharing personal items such as towels, toothbrushes, razors, or utensils. It is also advisable to stay home and seek medical attention when sick, and to follow the recommended vaccination schedule to prevent certain diseases. It is also beneficial to avoid or limit the contact with people or animals that are sick or infected, and to use protection when engaging in sexual activity. It is also helpful to boost the immune system by eating a balanced and nutritious diet, taking supplements such as vitamin C, zinc, and probiotics, and managing stress, sleep, and exercise.

Chapter 4: Natural Remedies for Common Immune Disorders

Natural Remedies for Common Immune Disorders

The body is shielded from dangerous invaders like bacteria, viruses, fungi, and parasites by the intricate network of cells, tissues, and organs that make up the immune system. The immune system also helps to regulate inflammation, which is a normal response to injury or infection. However, sometimes the immune system can malfunction and cause problems such as allergies, autoimmune diseases, chronic infections, and cancer. These are some of the common immune disorders that affect millions of people around the world.

Allergies: Allergies are hypersensitive reactions of the immune system to certain substances, such as pollen, dust, animal dander, food, or drugs. Allergies can cause symptoms such as sneezing, itching, runny nose, watery eyes, hives, rashes, swelling, or anaphylaxis. Some of the natural remedies that can help to reduce allergic reactions are:

Quercetin: One flavonoid with anti-inflammatory and antihistamine qualities is quercetin. It can help to inhibit the release of histamine, which is a chemical that triggers allergic symptoms. Quercetin can be found in foods such as apples, onions, berries, grapes, broccoli, and green tea, or taken as a supplement.

Bromelain: Bromelain is an enzyme that is derived from pineapple stems. It can help to reduce inflammation and swelling, and improve the absorption of quercetin. Bromelain can be taken as a supplement or eaten as fresh pineapple.

Nettle: Nettle is a herb that has anti-inflammatory and antihistamine effects. It can help to relieve nasal congestion, sneezing, and itching. Nettle can be consumed as a tincture, tea, or pill.

Autoimmune diseases: Autoimmune diseases are conditions where the immune system attacks the body's own tissues and organs, such as the joints, skin, thyroid, pancreas, or nervous system. Some of the common autoimmune diseases are rheumatoid arthritis, psoriasis, Hashimoto's thyroiditis, type 1 diabetes, and multiple sclerosis. Some of the natural remedies that can help to modulate the immune system and prevent or treat autoimmune diseases are:

Omega-3 fatty acids: Omega-3 fatty acids are essential fats that have anti-inflammatory and immunomodulatory effects. They can help to reduce the production of pro-inflammatory cytokines, which are molecules that promote inflammation and tissue damage. Omega-3 fatty acids can be found in foods such as fish, flaxseed, chia seeds, walnuts, and algae, or taken as a supplement.

Vitamin D: Vitamin D is a hormone that regulates the immune system and helps to prevent autoimmunity. Vitamin D can help to balance the activity of the T cells, which are a type of white blood cell that can either protect or attack the body.

Vitamin D can be obtained from sun exposure, foods such as fatty fish, egg yolks, mushrooms, and fortified dairy products, or taken as a supplement.

Curcumin: Curcumin is a compound that is extracted from turmeric, a spice that is widely used in Asian cuisine. Curcumin has anti-inflammatory and antioxidant properties. It can help to inhibit the activation of the nuclear factor-kappa B (NF-kB), which is a protein that controls the expression of genes that are involved in inflammation and autoimmunity. Curcumin can be taken as a supplement or added to food.

Chronic infections: Chronic infections are persistent or recurrent infections that are caused by microorganisms that evade or resist the immune system's defenses, such as bacteria, viruses, fungi, or parasites. Chronic infections can cause symptoms such as fever, fatigue, pain, inflammation, or organ dysfunction. Some of the natural remedies that can help to enhance the immune system's ability to fight chronic infections are:

Garlic: Garlic is a herb that has antimicrobial, antiviral, antifungal, and antiparasitic properties.

It can help to kill or inhibit the growth of various pathogens, such as Helicobacter pylori, Candida albicans, Escherichia coli, Staphylococcus aureus, and herpes simplex virus. Garlic can also stimulate the activity of the natural killer cells, which are a type of white blood cell that can destroy infected cells. Garlic can be eaten raw, cooked, or taken as a supplement.

Echinacea: Echinacea is a flower that has immunostimulant and anti-inflammatory effects. It can help to increase the production and function of the white blood cells, such as the macrophages, neutrophils, and lymphocytes, which are involved in the immune system's response to infections. Echinacea can also help to reduce the severity and duration of the symptoms of common colds and flu. Echinacea can be taken as a tea, capsule, or tincture.

Oregano oil: Oregano oil is an essential oil that is derived from the oregano plant. It has potent antimicrobial, antiviral, antifungal, and antiparasitic properties. It can help to kill or inhibit the growth of various pathogens, such as Streptococcus pneumoniae, Pseudomonas aeruginosa, Klebsiella pneumoniae, and

Giardia lamblia. Oregano oil can also help to boost the immune system's response to infections. Oregano oil can be taken as a capsule, diluted in water or oil, or applied topically.

What are the common immune disorders and their causes and symptoms?

Common Immune Disorders: Causes and Symptoms

The body's defense mechanism against pathogenic invaders including bacteria, viruses, fungi, and parasites is the immune system, a sophisticated network of cells, tissues, and organs. The immune system also helps to regulate inflammation, which is a normal response to injury or infection. However, sometimes the immune system can malfunction and cause problems such as allergies, autoimmune diseases, chronic infections, and cancer. These are some of the common immune disorders that affect millions of people around the world.

Allergies: Allergies are hypersensitive reactions of the immune system to certain substances, such as pollen, dust, animal dander, food, or drugs. The immune system mistakenly identifies these substances as foreign and dangerous, and produces antibodies to fight them. Histamine and other substances that induce allergy reactions are released as a result of this. The symptoms of allergies can vary depending on the type and severity of the reaction, but they may include sneezing, itching, runny nose, watery eyes, hives, rashes, swelling, or anaphylaxis. Anaphylaxis is a life-threatening condition that can cause difficulty breathing, low blood pressure, shock, or death. The causes of allergies are not fully understood, but they may involve genetic, environmental, and lifestyle factors.

Autoimmune diseases: Autoimmune diseases are conditions where the immune system attacks the body's own tissues and organs, such as the joints, skin, thyroid, pancreas, or nervous system. The immune system mistakenly recognizes these tissues and organs as foreign and harmful, and produces antibodies to destroy them.

This causes inflammation and tissue damage, which can lead to various symptoms and complications. The symptoms of autoimmune diseases can vary depending on the type and location of the affected tissue or organ, but they may include pain, stiffness, swelling, redness, heat, fatigue, fever, weight loss, hair loss, skin rashes, blisters, ulcers, dry eyes, dry mouth, numbness, tingling, weakness, paralysis, vision problems, hearing problems, cognitive problems, mood problems, or organ failure. The causes of autoimmune diseases are not fully understood, but they may involve genetic, environmental, hormonal, and infectious factors.

Chronic infections: Chronic infections are persistent or recurrent infections that are caused by microorganisms that evade or resist the immune system's defenses, such as bacteria, viruses, fungi, or parasites. The immune system is unable to eliminate these microorganisms completely, and they remain in the body for a long time, causing symptoms and complications. The symptoms of chronic infections can vary depending on the type and location of the infection, but they may include fever, fatigue, pain, inflammation, or organ dysfunction.

The causes of chronic infections may involve genetic, environmental, or lifestyle factors that weaken the immune system, or the ability of the microorganisms to adapt, mutate, or hide from the immune system.

Cancer: Cancer is a condition where the cells in the body grow and divide abnormally and uncontrollably, forming tumors or masses that can invade and damage the surrounding tissues and organs. Cancer can also spread to other parts of the body through the blood or lymphatic system, causing metastasis. The immune system plays a role in preventing and fighting cancer, by recognizing and eliminating abnormal or damaged cells, or by stimulating the production of natural killer cells, cytotoxic T cells, or antibodies that can target and destroy cancer cells. However, sometimes the immune system fails to do so, or the cancer cells evade or suppress the immune system's response, allowing the cancer to grow and progress. The symptoms of cancer can vary depending on the type and location of the cancer, but they may include lumps, bumps, moles, or growths that change in size, shape, color, or texture, pain, bleeding, bruising, swelling, weight loss, loss of appetite, fatigue, fever, night sweats, cough, shortness of breath, difficulty swallowing, hoarseness, nausea, vomiting, diarrhea, constipation, jaundice, or organ failure. The causes of cancer are not fully understood, but they may involve genetic, environmental, lifestyle, or infectious factors that damage the DNA of the cells, or interfere with the normal functioning of the immune system.

How to Prevent and Treat Common Immune Disorders Naturally

The body is shielded from dangerous invaders like bacteria, viruses, fungi, and parasites by the intricate network of cells, tissues, and organs that make up the immune system. The immune system also helps to regulate inflammation, which is a normal response to injury or infection. However, sometimes the immune system can malfunction and cause problems such as allergies, autoimmune diseases, chronic infections, and cancer. These are some of the common immune disorders that affect millions of people around the world.

Fortunately, there are some natural ways to prevent and treat these immune disorders, by supporting the immune system and restoring its balance and function. Here are some of them:

Diet: Diet plays a vital role in the immune system, as it provides the nutrients and energy that the immune cells need to perform their tasks. A healthy and balanced diet can help to prevent and treat immune disorders, by providing the essential vitamins, minerals, antioxidants, and phytochemicals that can modulate the immune system and reduce inflammation. Some of the foods that can boost the immune system are fruits, vegetables, nuts, seeds, legumes, whole grains, mushrooms, herbs, spices, and fermented foods. Some of the foods that can harm the immune system are processed foods, refined sugars, artificial sweeteners, trans fats, alcohol, and caffeine. Therefore, it is advisable to eat more of the former and less of the latter, and to avoid any food allergies or sensitivities that may trigger or worsen immune disorders.

Supplements: Supplements are substances that can provide additional or specific nutrients or compounds that may be lacking or insufficient in the diet, or that may have therapeutic effects on the immune system. Supplements can help to prevent and treat immune disorders, by enhancing the immune system's function and reducing inflammation. However, supplements should be used with caution and under the guidance of a health professional, as they may have side effects or interactions with other medications or supplements. Some of the supplements that can benefit the immune system are vitamin C, vitamin D, zinc, selenium, probiotics, omega-3 fatty acids, curcumin, quercetin, bromelain, echinacea, garlic, oregano oil, and astragalus.

Lifestyle: Lifestyle is another factor that can influence the immune system, as it affects the physical, mental, and emotional well-being of the individual. A healthy and balanced lifestyle can help to prevent and treat immune disorders, by reducing stress, improving sleep, increasing exercise, and maintaining hygiene.

Stress can weaken the immune system and increase inflammation, so it is important to find healthy ways to cope with stress, such as relaxation techniques, meditation, yoga, breathing exercises, hobbies, social support, counseling, or therapy. Sleep can restore the immune system and reduce inflammation, so it is recommended to get at least seven to eight hours of sleep per night, and to follow good sleep hygiene practices, such as having a regular sleep schedule, avoiding caffeine, alcohol, nicotine, and heavy meals before bedtime, keeping the bedroom dark, quiet, and comfortable, and avoiding the use of electronic devices before or during sleep. Exercise can improve blood circulation, oxygen delivery, and lymphatic drainage, which are all important for the immune system's function. Exercise can also reduce stress, improve mood, and enhance sleep quality, which can also boost the immune system. However, too much or too intense exercise can have the opposite effect, as it can cause physical and mental stress, inflammation, and tissue damage, which can impair the immune system and raise the possibility of illnesses and infections.

Therefore, it is advised to follow a moderate and balanced exercise routine, which includes aerobic, strength, and flexibility exercises, and to rest and recover adequately between workouts. Hygiene can prevent the exposure and transmission of harmful germs that can cause infections and diseases. Hygiene practices include washing the hands frequently and thoroughly with soap and water, especially before and after eating, after using the bathroom, after coughing, sneezing, or blowing the nose, and after touching potentially contaminated surfaces or objects. Hygiene also involves covering the mouth and nose with a tissue or elbow when coughing or sneezing, and disposing of the tissue properly. Hygiene also includes keeping the body, hair, nails, teeth, and clothes clean, and avoiding sharing personal items such as towels, toothbrushes, razors, or utensils. Hygiene also means staying home and seeking medical attention when sick, and following the recommended vaccination schedule to prevent certain diseases.

Natural Remedies for Colds, Flu, Allergies, Asthma, Autoimmune Diseases, and More

Colds, flu, allergies, asthma, and autoimmune diseases are some of the common immune disorders that affect millions of people around the world. They are caused by the malfunctioning of the immune system, which either fails to protect the body from harmful invaders, or attacks the body's own tissues and organs. These immune disorders can cause various symptoms and complications, such as fever, cough, sore throat, runny nose, congestion, sneezing, itching, wheezing, shortness of breath, rashes, hives, swelling, pain, inflammation, fatigue, weight loss, hair loss, organ dysfunction, or organ failure.

While there are conventional treatments available for these immune disorders, such as medications, inhalers, injections, or surgery, they may have side effects or limitations, and they may not address the root cause of the problem.

Therefore, many people are looking for natural remedies that can help to prevent and treat these immune disorders, by supporting the immune system and restoring its balance and function. Here are some of the natural remedies that can benefit the immune system and help to fight these immune disorders:

Honey: Honey is a natural sweetener that has antimicrobial, antiviral, anti-inflammatory, and antioxidant properties. It can help to soothe the throat, suppress the cough, kill or inhibit the growth of bacteria and viruses, reduce inflammation, and boost the immune system. Honey can be taken by itself, or mixed with lemon, ginger, or cinnamon, or added to tea, water, or milk. However, honey should not be given to children under one year of age, as it may contain botulinum spores that can cause infant botulism, a rare but serious condition that affects the nervous system.

Ginger: Ginger is a spice that has anti-inflammatory, antiviral, antifungal, and antioxidant effects. It can help to relieve nausea, vomiting, diarrhea, indigestion, gas, bloating, and cramps, and to stimulate the digestion and absorption of nutrients.

Ginger can also help to reduce inflammation, pain, and swelling, and to enhance the immune system's response to infections. Ginger can be taken as a tea, capsule, or tincture, or added to food, water, or juice.

Turmeric: Turmeric is a spice that has anti-inflammatory, antioxidant, antiviral, antifungal, and anticancer properties. It can help to inhibit the activation of the nuclear factor-kappa B (NF-kB), which is a protein that controls the expression of genes that are involved in inflammation and autoimmunity. Turmeric can also help to modulate the activity of the T cells, which are a type of white blood cell that can either protect or attack the body. Turmeric can also help to prevent or treat cancer, by inducing apoptosis, or programmed cell death, of the cancer cells, and by inhibiting angiogenesis, or the formation of new blood vessels that feed the tumors. Turmeric can be taken as a supplement or added to food, water, or milk. However, turmeric should be taken with black pepper, which contains piperine, a compound that can increase the absorption and bioavailability of curcumin, the active ingredient in turmeric.

Garlic: Garlic is a herb that has antimicrobial, antiviral, antifungal, and antiparasitic properties. It can help to kill or inhibit the growth of various pathogens, such as Helicobacter pylori, Candida albicans, Escherichia coli, Staphylococcus aureus, and herpes simplex virus. Garlic can also stimulate the activity of the natural killer cells, which are a type of white blood cell that can destroy infected cells. Garlic can also help to lower the blood pressure, cholesterol, and blood sugar levels, and to prevent or treat cardiovascular diseases, such as atherosclerosis, stroke, and heart attack. Garlic can be eaten raw, cooked, or taken as a supplement.

- Probiotics: Probiotics are beneficial bacteria that live in the gut and help to maintain the balance of the gut microbiota, which is the community of microorganisms that inhabit the digestive tract. The gut microbiota plays a crucial role in the immune system, as it helps to digest and absorb nutrients, produce vitamins and short-chain fatty acids, compete with pathogens, and modulate the immune system's function and response. Probiotics can help to prevent and treat immune disorders, by enhancing the gut barrier function, preventing the invasion and colonization of pathogens, reducing inflammation, and regulating the immune system's activity and tolerance. Probiotics can be found in fermented foods, such as yogurt, kefir, sauerkraut, kimchi, miso, tempeh, and kombucha, or taken as a supplement. However, probiotics should be chosen carefully, as different strains may have different effects, and some may not be suitable for certain conditions or individuals.

When to Seek Medical Help and What are the Conventional Treatments for Immune Disorders

Immune disorders are conditions where the immune system malfunctions and causes problems such as allergies, autoimmune diseases, chronic infections, and cancer. These immune disorders can affect various parts of the body and cause various symptoms and complications, such as fever, cough, sore throat, runny nose, congestion, sneezing, itching, wheezing, shortness of breath, rashes, hives, swelling, pain, inflammation, fatigue, weight loss, hair loss, organ dysfunction, or organ failure.

While there are some natural remedies that can help to prevent and treat these immune disorders, by supporting the immune system and restoring its balance and function, they may not be enough or effective for some cases or situations. Therefore, it is important to know when to seek medical help and what are the conventional treatments for these immune disorders.

When to Seek Medical Help

It is advisable to seek medical help for immune disorders in the following cases or situations:

When the symptoms are severe, persistent, recurrent, or interfere with daily activities or quality of life.

When the symptoms are accompanied by other signs of serious illness, such as high fever, difficulty breathing, chest pain, confusion, fainting, or bleeding.

When the symptoms do not improve or worsen after trying natural remedies or over-the-counter medications for a reasonable period of time.

When the symptoms are caused by a known or suspected allergen, and there is a risk of anaphylaxis, a life-threatening allergic reaction that can cause difficulty breathing, low blood pressure, shock, or death.

When the symptoms are caused by a known or suspected infection, there is a risk of complications, such as pneumonia, meningitis, sepsis, or organ failure.

When the symptoms are caused by a known or suspected autoimmune disease, and there is a risk of damage or dysfunction of the affected tissue or organ, such as the joints, skin, thyroid, pancreas, or nervous system.

When the symptoms are caused by a known or suspected cancer, and there is a risk of growth, invasion, or metastasis of the cancer cells to other parts of the body.

What are the Conventional Treatments

The conventional treatments for immune disorders may vary depending on the type, cause, and severity of the disorder, but they may include the following:

Medications: Medications are substances that can modify the immune system's function and response, or target the specific pathogens or cells that cause the disorder. Medications can help to prevent, treat, or control the symptoms and complications of immune disorders, by reducing inflammation, pain, swelling, itching, sneezing, coughing, congestion, or fever, or by killing or inhibiting the growth of bacteria, viruses, fungi, or parasites, or by destroying or suppressing the cancer cells. However, medications may have side effects or interactions with other medications or supplements, and they may not address the root cause of the problem. Some of the common medications for immune disorders are antihistamines, decongestants, corticosteroids, nonsteroidal anti-inflammatory drugs (NSAIDs), antibiotics, antivirals, antifungals, antiparasitics, immunosuppressants, immunomodulators, biologics, or chemotherapy.

Inhalers: Inhalers are devices that deliver medications directly to the lungs, where they can act on the airways and the respiratory system. Inhalers can help to prevent and treat immune disorders that affect the breathing, such as asthma, allergies, or chronic obstructive pulmonary disease (COPD). Inhalers can help to reduce inflammation, swelling, mucus production, and spasms of the airways, and to improve the airflow and oxygen delivery to the lungs. However, inhalers may have side effects or interactions with other medications or supplements, and they may not address the root cause of the problem. Some of the common inhalers for immune disorders are bronchodilators, corticosteroids, or combination inhalers.

Injections: Injections are methods of delivering medications or substances into the body through a needle or a syringe. Injections can help to prevent and treat immune disorders, by providing the immune system with the substances that it needs to function properly, or by modifying the immune system's function and response, or by targeting the specific pathogens or cells that cause the disorder. Injections can help to reduce inflammation, pain, swelling, itching, sneezing, coughing, congestion, or fever, or by killing or inhibiting the growth of bacteria, viruses, fungi, or parasites, or by destroying or suppressing the cancer cells. However, injections may have side effects or interactions with other medications or supplements, and they may not address the root cause of the problem. Some of the common injections for immune disorders are vaccines, immunoglobulins, allergen immunotherapy, or monoclonal antibodies.

- Surgery: Surgery is a procedure that involves the use of instruments or devices to remove, repair, or replace a part of the body that is affected by an immune disorder. Surgery can help to prevent and treat immune disorders, by removing the source of the problem, such as a tumor, an abscess, a cyst, or a foreign body, or by repairing or replacing the damaged or dysfunctional tissue or organ, such as a joint, a skin graft, a thyroid, a pancreas, or a nervous system. However, surgery may have risks or complications, such as bleeding, infection, scarring, or rejection, and it may not address the root cause of the problem. Some of the common surgeries for immune disorders are excision, drainage, biopsy, arthroplasty, skin grafting, thyroidectomy, pancreas transplantation, or neurosurgery.

Conclusion

A summary of the main points and key takeaways from the book

The body is shielded from dangerous invaders like bacteria, viruses, fungi, and parasites by the intricate network of cells, tissues, and organs that make up the immune system. The immune system also helps to regulate inflammation, which is a normal response to injury or infection. However, sometimes the immune system can malfunction and cause problems such as allergies, autoimmune diseases, chronic infections, and cancer.

The book "How to Boost Immune System Naturally" provides practical and evidence-based tips on how to strengthen the immune system and prevent or treat these immune disorders, by following a healthy and balanced diet, lifestyle, and supplementation. The book covers the following topics:

The role and function of the immune system, and the factors that can affect its performance and balance.

The common immune disorders, their causes, symptoms, and complications, and how they can be diagnosed and treated with conventional and natural methods.

The foods that can boost the immune system, such as fruits, vegetables, nuts, seeds, legumes, whole grains, mushrooms, herbs, spices, and fermented foods, and the nutrients and antioxidants that they provide, such as vitamin C, vitamin D, zinc, selenium, probiotics, omega-3 fatty acids, curcumin, quercetin, bromelain, echinacea, garlic, oregano oil, and astragalus.

The foods that can harm the immune system, such as processed foods, refined sugars, artificial sweeteners, trans fats, alcohol, and caffeine, and the inflammation and oxidative stress that they cause, and how to avoid or limit them, and to identify and eliminate any food allergens or sensitivities that may trigger or worsen immune disorders.

The supplements that can support the immune system, such as vitamin C, vitamin D, zinc, selenium, probiotics, omega-3 fatty acids, curcumin, quercetin, bromelain, echinacea, garlic, oregano oil, and astragalus, and how to choose, use, and combine them safely and effectively, and under the guidance of a health professional.

The lifestyle factors that can influence the immune system, such as stress, sleep, exercise, and hygiene, and how to manage them for optimal immune health, such as finding healthy ways to cope with stress, getting enough and quality sleep, following a moderate and balanced exercise routine, and practicing good hygiene habits.

The natural remedies that can help to prevent and treat common immune disorders, such as honey, ginger, turmeric, garlic, probiotics, and inhalers, and how to use them properly and appropriately, and in conjunction with conventional treatments if needed.

The book **"How to Boost Immune System Naturally"** is a comprehensive and informative guide that can help anyone who wants to improve their immune health and prevent or treat common immune disorders, by following a natural and holistic approach that is based on scientific research and clinical experience. The book is written in a clear and easy-to-understand language, and provides practical and realistic advice, examples, and recipes that can be easily implemented and adapted to individual needs and preferences.

You have just learned about some natural strategies to boost your immune system, such as eating healthy foods, getting enough sleep, exercising regularly, and managing stress. These strategies can help you prevent or fight off infections, diseases, and illnesses. But knowing is not enough. You need to take action and apply these strategies to your daily life.

Here are some ways you can start implementing these natural strategies today:

Eat more fruits and vegetables. They are rich in vitamins, minerals, antioxidants, and phytochemicals that can enhance your immune system.

Try to eat a variety of colors and types of produce every day. Some examples are citrus fruits, berries, leafy greens, carrots, broccoli, garlic, and ginger.

Make sure you sleep for seven or eight hours every night. Your immune system needs to sleep in order to work correctly. It helps your body repair and regenerate cells, produce antibodies, and fight inflammation. Lack of sleep can impair your immune response and make you more susceptible to infections.

Exercise moderately for at least 30 minutes a day, five days a week. Exercise can improve your blood circulation, reduce stress, and strengthen your muscles and bones. It can also stimulate your immune system by increasing the activity of natural killer cells and macrophages, which can destroy pathogens and infected cells.

Manage your stress levels. Stress can weaken your immune system by releasing hormones such as cortisol and adrenaline, which can suppress your immune cells and increase inflammation. Chronic stress can also affect your mood, sleep, appetite, and mental health.

To cope with stress, you can try relaxation techniques such as meditation, yoga, breathing exercises, or hobbies that you enjoy.

By following these natural strategies, you can boost your immune system and protect your health. You can also benefit from other positive outcomes, such as improved energy, mood, and well-being. Don't wait any longer. Start taking action today and see the difference for yourself. You have nothing to lose and everything to gain. Your immune system will be appreciative.

A list of additional resources and references for further reading and learning

A Lifestyle Action Plan for Strengthening Your Body's Defenses by Dr. J. K. Evans. This book provides practical advice and tips on how to improve your immunity through diet, supplements, exercise, and stress management. You can find it on [Amazon] or [Goodreads].

Thank you for buying this book and reading it until the end. I hope you enjoyed it and learned something valuable from it. I appreciate your interest and support for this topic.

If you liked this book, please consider leaving a positive review on [Amazon] or [Goodreads]. Your feedback is very important for me and other potential readers. It will help me improve my writing and reach more people who can benefit from this book.

To leave a review, you can follow these steps:

Go to the [Amazon] or [Goodreads] page of this book. Select the "Write a review" or "Write a customer review" button.

Rate the book from one to five stars and write a brief comment about what you liked or disliked about the book.

Submit your review and share it with your friends and family.

Thank you for your time and generosity. I hope you have a wonderful day and stay healthy and happy!